CBT for Children, Adolescents, and Adults

Strategies for Managing Anti-Personality, Disruptive Behaviour, Anti-Social Personality, Avoidant Personality, Oppositional Defiant & Conduct Disorders

Dr. Dale Pheragh

Table of Contents

CBT FOR CHILDREN, ADOLESCENTS, AND ADULTS 1

INTRODUCTION 6

CHAPTER 1 9

What is Conduct Disorder? 9
- What Causes Conduct Disorder? 9
- Who is Suffering from Conduct Disorder? 10
- What are the symptoms of Conduct Disorder? 11
- How is Conduct Disorder diagnosed? 13
- Treatment for Conduct Disorder 14
- Prevention of Conduct Disorder in Children 15

CHAPTER 2 17

What does having Conduct Disorder mean for a Person 17
- What effect can this have on others? 17
- What are the longer-term ramifications of Conduct Disorder? 19
- What are the types of help you need there? 20

CHAPTER 3 25

Signs of Conduct Disorder 25
- Types of Conduct Disorder 26

CHAPTER 4 29

Causes of Conduct Disorder 29
Who is suffering from Conduct Disorder? 30

CHAPTER 5 31

The Characteristics of Conduct Disorder 31

CHAPTER 6 36

Diagnosis 36

Treatment...*36*

CHAPTER 7 ....**39**

WHAT HELP IS DESIGNED FOR CONDUCT DISORDER? 39

Home-Based Help *40*

School-Based Help *41*

Community-Based Help *42*

CHAPTER 8 ....**44**

ASSISTING YOUR ADOLESCENT WITH CONDUCT DISORDER 44

Adolescent Conduct Disorder - statistics and facts *45*

How to Proceed When Things Escalate *55*

Caring for Yourself *58*

CHAPTER 9 ....**60**

TANTRUM 60

What can cause a tantrum? *60*

What may I do when my child is having a Tantrum? *61*

What may I do to avoid temper tantrums? *63*

Where may I get help? *64*

CHAPTER 10 ....**65**

PERSONALITY DISORDERS: HELPFUL INFORMATION TO THE 10 DIFFERENT KINDS 65

CHAPTER 11 ....**76**

AVOIDANT PERSONALITY DISORDER 76

WHAT CAUSES AVOIDANT PERSONALITY DISORDER? 77

AVOIDANT PERSONALITY DISORDER SYMPTOMS 78

What is a Cluster C Personality Disorder? *79*

Treatment for Avoidant Personality Disorder *81*

CHAPTER 12 ....**84**

ANTISOCIAL PERSONALITY DISORDER..84

SYMPTOMS 86

CAUSES 87

TREATMENT 87
    At what Age can Antisocial Personality Disorder be Diagnosed? 89
    How to Cope whenever a Cherished One has Antisocial Personality Disorder 90

CHAPTER 13 92

OPPOSITIONAL DEFIANT DISORDER 92
WHAT CAN CAUSE OPPOSITIONAL DEFIANT DISORDER? 92
    What are the symptoms of Oppositional Defiant Disorder? 94
    How is Oppositional Defiant Disorder Diagnosed? 95
    Treatment for Oppositional Defiant Disorder 96
    Avoidance of Oppositional Defiant Disorder in Children 98

CHAPTER 14 100

DISRUPTIVE BEHAVIOUR DISORDERS 100
    Oppositional Defiant Disorder 101
    ODD and Conduct Disorder: What things to look for 103
    Treatment 105

Copyright © 2020 Dr. Dale Pheragh

All rights reserved. No part of this publication may be reproduced, distributed, or transmitted in any form or by any means, including photocopying, recording, or other electronic or mechanical methods, without the prior written permission of the publisher, except in the case of brief quotations embodied in critical reviews and specific other non-commercial uses permitted by copyright law.

ISBN: 978-1-63750-190-0

Introduction

The CBT guide for Children and Adolescents gives you the resources to help the children in your life handle their daily obstacles with ease.

Inside this workbook you'll find hundreds of worksheets, exercises, and activities to help treat:

- ✓ *Ideal Solution for Anti-Personality Disorder*
- ✓ *Tantrum,*
- ✓ *Disruptive Behaviour Disorder,*
- ✓ *Anti-Social Personality Disorder,*
- ✓ *Avoidant Personality Disorder,*
- ✓ *Oppositional Defiant Disorder & Conduct Disorders*
- ✓ *Conduct Disorders*

Written by a doctor with decades of experience working with kids, teens, adults and these practical and easy-to-use therapy tools are vital to teaching people how to cope with and overcome their deepest struggles. Step-by-step, you'll see how the best strategies from cognitive behavioral therapy are adapted for children.

Conduct disorder, sometimes diagnosed in child years, that is seen as antisocial actions which violate the privileges of others and age-appropriate sociable standards and guidelines. Antisocial behaviors can include irresponsibility, delinquent acts (such as truancy or operating away), breaking the rights of others (such as robbery), and physical hostility toward pets or others (such as assault or rape). These behaviors sometimes happen collectively; however, one or several might occur with no other(s).

Conduct Disorder is a significant behavioral and emotional disorder that may appear in children and teenagers. A kid with this disorder may screen the design of disruptive and violent behavior and also have problems following guidelines.

It isn't uncommon for children and teenagers to have behavior-related problems sometime throughout their development. However, the behavior is known as to be always a Conduct Disorder when it's long-lasting, so when it violates the privileges of others, it will go against accepted norms of behavior and disrupt the child's or families' everyday living.

A definitive guide to recognizing what factors cause defiant episodes in children, adolescents, & adults and tips to help identify when and where these problematic behaviors are likely to occur. Containing tools to increase positive behaviors, this is an ideal resource for therapists, educators and parents.

- ✓ Non-medication approaches to ODD, ADHD, anxiety, mood and disruptive disorders
- ✓ Exercises, assessments, guidelines and case studies
- ✓ Crisis Prevention and Intervention
- ✓ Safety Plans and Risk Evaluations
- ✓ Evaluate and Treat Co-morbidity

Tools and Strategies for:
- ✓ Noncompliance
- ✓ Nagging
- ✓ Yelling/screaming
- ✓ Bullying
- ✓ Panic/anxiety reactions
- ✓ Lack of follow-through
- ✓ Running away
- ✓ Tantrum.

Chapter 1
What is Conduct Disorder?

Conduct Disorder is a behavior disorder, sometimes diagnosed in youth, that is seen as an antisocial habit which violates the privileges of others and age-appropriate public standards and guidelines. Antisocial behaviors can include irresponsibility, delinquent behaviors (such as truancy or working away), breaking the rights of others (such as fraud), and physical hostility toward pets or others (such as assault or rape). These behaviors sometimes take place jointly; however, one or several might occur with no other(s).

What Causes Conduct Disorder?

The conditions that donate to the introduction of Conduct Disorder are believed to be multifactorial, and therefore, many factors give to this. Neuropsychological testing shows that children with Conduct Disorders seem to have impairment in the frontal lobe of the mind that inhibits their capability to plan, avoid damage, and study from negative encounters. Childhood character is considered to have a genetic basis indeed. Children who are believed to have a complicated role indeed will develop behavior problems. Children from disadvantaged, dysfunctional, and disorganized home conditions will develop Conduct Disorders, though it is available in all socioeconomic groupings. Cultural issues and peer group rejection have been found to donate to delinquency. The low socioeconomic position has been associated with Conduct Disorders. Children exhibiting delinquent and intense behaviors have distinctive cognitive and mental profiles in comparison with children with other mental health issues and control organizations. All the possible adding factors impact how children connect to other people.

Who is Suffering from Conduct Disorder?

The disorder is more prevalent in boys than in girls. Children with Conduct Disorders frequently have other psychiatric problems as well that may donate to the introduction of the Conduct Disorder. The prevalence of

Conduct Disorders has increased over recent years across races, civilizations, and socioeconomic groupings.

What are the symptoms of Conduct Disorder?

Most symptoms observed in children with Conduct Disorder also occur sometimes in children without this disorder. However, in children with Conduct Disorder, these symptoms happen more often and hinder learning, school modification, and, sometimes, with the child's interactions with others.

Listed below are the most typical symptoms of Conduct Disorder. However, each young one may experience the symptoms differently. The four main sets of behaviors are the following:

- **Aggressive conduct:**

    Aggressive Conduct causes or threatens physical injury to others and could include the pursuing:
    - ✓ Intimidating behavior.
    - ✓ Bullying.
    - ✓ Physical fights.

- ✓ Cruelty to others or animals.
- ✓ Usage of a tool(s).
- ✓ Forcing someone into sex, rape, or molestation

- **Destructive conduct:**
Destructive Conduct may include the following: Vandalism, intentional damage to property.
- *Deceitfulness:* Deceitful behavior can include the following;
    - ✓ Lying.
    - ✓ Theft.
    - ✓ Shoplifting.
    - ✓ Delinquency.
- *Violation of guidelines:* Violation of regular rules of Conduct or age-appropriate norms can include the following:
    - ✓ Truancy (failing to attend college).
    - ✓ Running away.
    - ✓ Pranks.
    - ✓ Mischief.

- ✓ Very early sex

The symptoms of Conduct Disorder look like other medical ailments or behavioral problems. Always seek advice from your son or daughter's doctor for a medical diagnosis.

How is Conduct Disorder diagnosed?

A kid psychiatrist or a professional mental doctor usually diagnoses Conduct Disorders in children. A detailed background of the child's behavior from parents and instructors, observations of the child's behavior, and, sometimes, emotional testing donates to the medical diagnosis. Parents who notice symptoms of Conduct Disorder in the youngster or teenager can help by seeking an assessment and treatment early. Early treatment could prevent future problems.

Further, Conduct Disorder often coexists with other mental health disorders, including feeling disorders, anxiousness disorders, posttraumatic stress disorder, drug abuse, attention-deficit/hyperactivity disorder, and learning disorders, increasing the necessity for early analysis and treatment. Check with your child's doctor to find out more.

Treatment for Conduct Disorder

Specific treatment for children with Conduct Disorders will be dependent on your son or daughter's doctor predicated on:

- Your son or daughter's age, general health, and health background.
- The extent of your son or daughter's symptoms.
- Your son or daughter's tolerance for specific medications or therapies.
- Anticipations for the span of the condition.
- Your opinion or preference.
- Treatment can include:

- ***Cognitive-behavioural approaches:*** The purpose of cognitive-behavioural therapy is to boost problem resolving skills, communication skills, impulse control, and anger management skills.

- *Family therapy:* Family therapy is often centred on making changes within the family system, such as enhancing communication skills and family relationships.

- *Peer group therapy*: Peer group therapy is often centred on developing public skills and social skills.

- *Medication:* Without considered effective in dealing with Conduct Disorder, medication can be utilized if other symptoms or disorders can be found attentive to medication.

Prevention of Conduct Disorder in Children

Much like Oppositional Defiant Disorder (ODD), some experts think that a developmental series of encounters occur in the introduction of Conduct Disorder. This series may begin with inadequate parenting practices, accompanied by educational failing, and poor peer connections. These encounters then often lead to depressed disposition and participation in a deviant peer group. Other experts, however, think that many factors, including child misuse, genetic susceptibility, the background of educational failure, brain harm, and distressing experience, impact the manifestation of Conduct Disorder. Early recognition and treatment into negative family and interpersonal encounters may help disrupt the introduction of the series of battles that lead to more disruptive and intense behaviors.

Chapter 2
What does having Conduct Disorder mean for a Person

Children with a Conduct Disorder get involved with more violent physical battles and may steal or lie, with no indication of remorse or guilt when they are found out. They won't follow the rules and could begin to break regulations. They may start to stay out forever and play truancy from college throughout the day.

Teenagers with Conduct Disorder could also take dangers with their health insurance and safety by firmly taking unlawful drugs or having unprotected sexual activity.

What effect can this have on others?

Conduct Disorder can result in a great deal of stress to children, family members, universities, and local areas. Children who behave, such as this, will often think it is hard to socialize and have trouble understanding interpersonal situations.

Even though they could be quite shiny, they'll not prosper at school and tend to be near the bottom level of the course. Inside, the young person may be feeling they are worthless, and they cannot do anything right. It's quite common to allow them to show anger and also to blame others for his or her difficulties if indeed they have no idea how to improve for the better.

What can cause Oppositional Defiant Disorder/Conduct Disorder?

There is absolutely no single reason behind Conduct Disorder. We are starting to understand that there are various possible reasons which businesses lead to Conduct Disorder. A kid may become more likely to develop an Oppositional Defiant Disorder/Conduct Disorder if indeed they:

- Have specific genes resulting in antisocial behavior.
- Have difficulties learning good sociable and acceptable behaviors.
- Have a hard temperament.
- Have learning or reading difficulties, which makes

it hard to allow them to understand and be a part of lessons; it is then possible for these to get fed up, feel ridiculous, and misbehave.

- Are depressed.
- Have already been bullied or abused.

Are 'hyperactive' - this causes problems with self-control, attending to, and following guidelines.

- Are participating with other awkward teenagers and medication misuse.
- *Other factors:* Boys will have behavioral problems and Conduct Disorder than women. Parenting factors, including discipline issues and family disorganization - parents will often make things worse giving too little focus on good behavior, always being too quick to criticize or when you are also versatile about the guidelines rather than supervising their children.

What are the longer-term ramifications of Conduct Disorder?

A person showing signs of Conduct Disorder young is

much more likely to be male, have Attention Deficit Hyperactivity Disorder (ADHD), and lower intelligence (general learning disability or specific difficulties in reading). The sooner the issues start, the bigger the chance of the young person finding himself being associated with assault and criminal functions. This might also be related to companionship groupings, gangs and the use of unlawful substances.

What are the types of help you need there?

Early diagnosis of Conduct Disorder and other related difficulties is essential to provide your child with a much better opportunity for improvement and expectations from the future.

With regard to the severity of the problem, the procedure can be offered across different settings - for example, at home or in educational and community settings. The assistance provided depends on the child's development, age group, and circumstances.

Involving and helping the family is vital. Focusing on advantages and determining any specific trouble spots for the young person, such as learning problems, can enhance the results for teenagers with Conduct Disorders. Help for behavioral problems can involve helping the young person to increase their positive, friendly behaviors, and controlling their destructive antisocial behaviors.

- **Home-based help**

It could be problematic for parents and carers when the youngster has Oppositional Defiant Disorder or Conduct problems. You might dread your child and feel ashamed or even ashamed of your son or daughter's situation.

You might feel helpless and unsure of how to control it.

As a mother or father, it could be easy to ignore your son or daughter when they may have been good and pay focus on them when they are misbehaving. As time passes, the child discovers that they only get attention when they may be breaking the guidelines. Most children, including teens, need a great deal of attention using their parents and could be unsure ways to get this. Perhaps remarkably, they appear to prefer the furious or critical focus on being overlooked. It is simple to observe how, as time passes, a vicious group can be setup.

With children, it can be beneficial if discipline is fair and constant as well as for parents/carers to agree about how to take care of their child's behavior and provide positive praise and love. This is difficult to control alone with no support of others, and many parents/carers require extra help.

Parenting organizations can help you on how to gain access to the support you will need, and share encounters with other people who are facing similar issues with their children. These groupings can offer to learn, assisting you in encouraging positive behavior in your son or daughter.

- **School-based help**

Many teenagers with behavioral problems struggle at school, which is a way to obtain distress. School staff can help concentrate on positive behaviors and reinforce work occurring at home and locally. Teenagers with behavioral problems often need help with cultural skills, and school might be able to offer this. Some children need specific classroom support and evaluation of learning issues. When the problems are severe, some children may need to be relocated to individual educational placements or institutions where their behavioral issues can be handled.

- **Community-based help**

If the behavioral problems are severe and persistent or a Conduct Disorder is suspected, ask your GP for advice.

Antisocial behaviors are generally observed in specialist services. If expert help is necessary, the GP can make a recommendation to your neighborhood Child and Adolescent Mental Health Service (CAMHS). This specialist team will continue to work as well as you, the institution, and other community organizations to aid you as well as your child.

Specialists can helpfully assess what's leading to the problem and suggesting practical means of enhancing the problematic behavior. They can also offer evaluation and treatment of other conditions that may appear at precisely the same time, such as major depression, panic, and hyperactivity. The treatment can include social skills groups, behavioral therapy, and talking therapy. These therapies can help the kid to appropriately exhibit themselves in various situations, and manage their anger better.

Chapter 3
Signs of Conduct Disorder

Conduct Disorder extends beyond healthy teenage rebellion. It entails serious behavior issues that will probably increase alarm among educators, parents, peers, and other adults.

To be able to be eligible for a diagnosis of Conduct Disorder, children must exhibit at least three symptoms before a year or with at least one sign before half a year:

- Hostility toward people and animals.
- Often bullies threaten or intimidate others.
- Often initiates physical fights.
- Has used a tool that might lead to serious harm.
- Physical cruelty to the people.
- Physical cruelty to animals.
- Stealing while confronting a victim.
- Forced sex.
- Property Destruction.
- Deliberate open fire setting.
- Other destruction of property.

- Deceptiveness or Theft.
- Breaking or getting into a residence, car, or building.
- Lying for personal gain.
- Stealing without confronting the owner (such as shoplifting).
- Serious Guideline Violation
- Staying out during the night or being truant before the age group of 13 years
- Has tried to escape from their homes overnight at least twice
- Is often missing from college, beginning before the age group of 13

Types of Conduct Disorder

The DSM-5, which is utilized to diagnose mental illnesses, distinguishes between Conduct Disorder with or without limited prosocial emotions. People with inadequate prosocial feelings are seen as too little remorse, are callous, and without empathy.

They may be unconcerned about their performance at school or work and also have shallow feelings. When present, their psychological expressions enable you to manipulate others.

Conduct Disorder Impairs a Child's Functioning

Conduct Disorder isn't only a problem for caregivers-it impairs a child's capability to function. Children with Conduct Disorder misbehave a lot that their education is affected. They often receive regular disciplinary action from instructors and could be truant. Children with Conduct Disorder may be at an increased risk of falling or shedding out of college.

Children with Conduct Disorder likewise have weak associations. They battle to develop and keep maintaining friendships. Their human relationships with family usually suffer because of the intensity of their behavior.

Adolescents with Conduct Disorder are also much more likely to have legal problems. Drug abuse, violent behavior, and a disregard for regulations can lead to incarceration.

They could also be at an increased threat of sexually transmitted infections. Studies also show that teens with Conduct Disorder will have multiple intimate partners, and they're less inclined to use protection.

Chapter 4
Causes of Conduct Disorder

Conduct Disorder identifies a variety of problems and does not have any clear, solitary purpose. It's been associated with:

- Child misuse and neglect.
- Drug or alcoholic beverages mistreatment by parents.
- Family conflict.
- Harsh or inconsistent discipline.
- Interpersonal problems and rejection by peers.
- Exposure to assault or other trauma.
- Hereditary factors, including Antisocial Personality Disorder in parents.
- Poverty.
- **Brain abnormalities** - Neuroimaging studies suggest that children with Conduct Disorder may involve some functional anomalies using regions of the mind. The pre-frontal cortex (which impacts view), and the limbic system (which affects

emotional reactions), may be impaired.

- ***Genetics*** - Studies suggest that anti-social behavior is approximately 50 percent inheritable. Experts aren't sure what hereditary components donate to Conduct Disorder.
- ***Sociable issues*** - Poverty, disorganized neighborhoods, junior colleges, family breakdown, parental psychopathology, harsh parenting, and insufficient supervision are strongly correlated with Conduct Disorder.
- ***Cognitive deficits*** - Low IQ, poor verbal skills, and impairment in professional functioning could make children more susceptible to Conduct Disorder.

Who is suffering from Conduct Disorder?

The disorder is more prevalent in boys than in girls. Children with Conduct Disorders frequently have other psychiatric problems as well that may donate to the introduction of the Conduct Disorder. The prevalence of Conduct Disorders has increased over recent years across races, ethnicities, and socioeconomic organizations.

Chapter 5

The Characteristics of Conduct Disorder

A number of the typical behaviors of a kid with CD can include:

- Refusal to obey parents or other authority figures, i.e., Truancy
- An inclination to use drugs, including cigarette and alcoholic beverages, at an extremely early age.
- Insufficient empathy for others.
- Spiteful and vengeful behavior.
- Being aggressive to animals.
- Being aggressive to the people, including bullying and physical or sexual abuse.
- A tendency to hold out in gangs.
- Keenness to begin physical fights.
- Using weapons in physical fights.
- Lying.
- Law-breaking behavior such as stealing, deliberately light fires, breaking into homes, shoplifting, intimate abuse, and vandalism.

- A tendency to hightail it.
- Learning difficulties.
- Low self-esteem.
- Suicidal tendencies.

The hyperlink to other behavioral disorders:
A kid who eventually develops Conduct Disorder is usually irritable and temperamental during babyhood - although most challenging infants do not develop Conduct Disorder. The milder Oppositional Defiant Disorder (ODD) often evolves before CD. Regular defiance, hostility, and a hair-trigger temper are typical characteristics of ODD.

Around one-third of children with Conduct Disorder likewise, have Attention Deficit Hyperactivity Disorder (ADHD). One in five children with Conduct Disorder is depressed. Conduct Disorder is typically diagnosed when the kid is between 10 and 16 years, with males generally diagnosed at a young age than ladies.

The influence of the family:

The sources of disruptive behavior disorders are unfamiliar, but researchers have discovered that all children with CD have family difficulties; a child's family life is a robust risk factor for most. A number of the factors that increase a child's threat of developing Conduct Disorder include:

- Parents who do not have collection limits on the child's behavior.
- Parents who do not continue with effects for unacceptable behavior (for example, a mother or father may threaten to withdraw TV for night time but not continue when the child's behavior doesn't change).
- Insufficient parental monitoring of the child's or adolescent's whereabouts.
- Unsatisfied family life numerous arguments.
- Poverty.
- Large family.
- Aggressive parenting, particularly from the daddy.
- Marital conflict.

- Domestic violence.
- Parents with a mental medical condition.
- Parents who get excited about law-breaking behavior.
- Child abuse.
- Surviving in institutionalized care and attention.

Other factors:

Other factors that may donate to the introduction of Conduct Disorder or exacerbate the characteristics of the disorder include:

- Gender - males are doubly likely as girls to have CD.
- Peer group.
- Substance misuse.
- Mood disorders.
- Learning difficulties.
- Post-Traumatic Stress Disorder (PTSD).
- Depression.
- Oppositional Defiant Disorder (ODD).
- Attention Deficit Hyperactivity Disorder (ADHD).

- Brain damage.

Possible consequences:

Untreated, a few of the possible outcomes in adulthood for children with Conduct Disorder include:

- Mental health issues, including personality disorders.
- Depression.
- Alcoholism.
- Drug dependency.
- Law-breaking lifestyle.

Chapter 6
Diagnosis

CD stocks similarities with ODD and ADHD, making diagnosis difficult. Conduct Disorder must be expertly diagnosed by a kid or adolescent psychologist, child psychiatrist, or pediatrician specializing in the region of behavior disorders.

The professional can make their assessment predicated on observation and interviews with the parents, the adolescent, and teachers. The adolescent's behavior is in comparison to a checklist in the Diagnostic and Statistical Manual of Mental Disorders from the American Psychiatric Association. If sufficient requirements are fulfilled, an analysis of Conduct Disorder can be produced.

Treatment

One of the most significant difficulties in treating a kid with Conduct Disorder is to overcome their mistrust of others, particularly expert numbers. The child's unwillingness to check out any rules must be taken into consideration. It might take a while to unravel the many factors that donate to the child's behavior and take appropriate action.

Treatment depends on the average person but can include:
- Behavior therapy.
- Cognitive Behavioural Therapy (CBT).
- Anger management.
- Stress management.
- Sociable skills training.
- Special education program.
- Mother or father management training.
- Family therapy.
- Multisystemic therapy.
- Integrated approach by family, teachers, and other carers.
- Management of any co-existing problems.
- Medication (in case there is a co-existing depressive disorder or ADHD).

Where you might get help

- Your physician (for a recommendation to a specialized service)
- Child or adolescent psychologist.

What to remember

Conduct Disorder (Conduct Disorder) is a behavioral problem in children, which might involve hostility and law-breaking tendencies. Behaviors include aversion to pets and other folks, and law-breaking activities such as deliberately light fires, shoplifting, and vandalism. The child's family life is a substantial risk element in the introduction of the CD.

Treatment plans include behavior therapy, psychotherapy, mother or father management training, and functional family therapy.

Chapter 7

What Help is Designed for Conduct Disorder?

Early diagnosis of Conduct Disorder and other related difficulties is essential to provide your child with a much better opportunity for improvements and expect the future.

With regard to the severity of the problem, the procedure can be offered across different settings, for example, at home or in educational and community settings. The assistance provided depends on the child's development, age, and circumstances.

Involving and helping the family is vital. Focusing on talents and determining any specific trouble spots for the young person, such as learning complications, can enhance the final results for teenagers with Conduct Disorders.

Help for behavioral problems can involve helping the young person to increase their positive, friendly behaviors, and controlling their destructive antisocial behaviors.

Home-Based Help

It could be problematic for parents and carers when the youngster has oppositional or has Conduct problems. You might dread your child and feel uncomfortable or even ashamed of your child's situation. You might feel helpless and uncertain of how to control it.

As a mother or father, it could be easy to ignore your son or daughter when they may be being kind, and pay focus on them when these are misbehaving. As time passes, the child discovers that they only get attention when they may be breaking guidelines. Most children, including teens, need a great deal of care of their parents and could be unsure ways to get this. Perhaps amazingly, they appear to prefer an irritated or critical focus on being ignored. You can see how, as time passes, a 'vicious routine' can be created.

With children, it can be beneficial if discipline is fair and constant as well as for parents/carers to agree about how to take care of their child's behavior and provide positive praise and love. Understandably, this is difficult to control alone with no support of others, and many parents/carers require extra help.

Parenting organizations can enable you to gain access to the support you will need and share encounters with other people who are experiencing an identical situation using their children. These groupings can offer trained in assisting support you in motivating positive behavior in your son or daughter.

School-Based Help

Many teenagers with behavioral problems struggle at school, which is a way to obtain distress. School personnel can help concentrate on positive behaviors and strengthen work occurring at home and locally.

Teenagers with behavioral problems often need help with public skills, and schools might be able to offer this. Some children need specific class support and evaluation of learning troubles. When the issues are severe, some children may be positioned in individual educational placements or academic institutions because of their behavioral problems.

Community-Based Help

If the behavioral problems are severe and persistent or a Conduct Disorder is suspected, ask your GP for advice.

Antisocial behaviors are generally observed in specialist services. If expert help is needed, they'll make a recommendation to your neighborhood child and adolescent mental health service (CAMHS). This specialist team will continue to work as well as you, college, and other community organizations to aid you as well as your child.

Specialists can helpfully assess what's leading to the problem and suggesting practical means of enhancing the problematic behavior. They can also offer evaluation and treatment of other conditions which may appear at the same time, such as melancholy, stress and anxiety, and hyperactivity.

The treatment can include social skills groups, behavioral therapy, and talking therapy. These therapies can help the kid to appropriately go to town in various situations and manage their anger better.

Chapter 8
Assisting Your Adolescent with Conduct Disorder

Frequent acting away, cruelty to the people or pets, defiance, and intense behavior are just some of the indicators of Conduct Disorder in children and young adults. While a few of these behaviors can be alarming to parents, they can likewise have severe implications for your teenager, including getting suspended or expelled from college or getting in a juvenile detention service.

Fortunately, medicine in the early stages can employ a positive effect on teens with Conduct Disorder. However, first, you should know what things to look for, and the steps to try to ensure your young has got the help she or he needs.

This brief guide was created to help you identify the signs and know very well what steps to take if you were to think your child has Conduct Disorder.

Adolescent Conduct Disorder - statistics and facts

1. Conduct Disorder is almost doubly common in men than females - in the overall population, around 6 to 16% of kids have Conduct Disorder, while somewhere within 2% to 9% own it.
2. Conduct Disorder is much more likely to build up in youngsters who grow up in cities than in rural areas.
3. Conduct Disorder influences around 1% to 4% of youngsters between the age groups of 9 and 17.
4. In mental health settings, Conduct Disorder is one of the most commonly diagnosed psychiatric disorders among children and adolescents.
5. Conduct Disorder begins in years as a child or adolescence - "child-onset" develops before age group 10 and has an even worse prognosis than "adolescent-onset."
6. Teenagers with adolescent-onset Conduct Disorder

are less inclined to be identified as having antisocial personality after age group 18 than people that have child-onset Conduct Disorder
7. Treatment for Conduct Disorder is much more likely to work if started early.
8. Disruptive behavior disorder is another name for Conduct Disorder

Co-occurring Disorders

Other mental health disorders that often exist before or co-occur with Conduct Disorder include:
- Attention-Deficit Hyperactivity Disorder (ADHD).
- Post-Traumatic Stress Disorder (PTSD).
- Oppositional Defiant Disorder (ODD).
- Depression.
- Anxiety.
- Material use disorders.

    Risk factors for Conduct Disorder include:
- A brief history of abuse or neglect.
- Any background of trauma.
- Genetic predisposition.
- Failing in school.

- A traumatic brain injury

Looking for and Realizing the Signals of Perform Disorder

To get your child the assistance he or she needs as soon as possible, which is vital with Conduct Disorder, you should know what things to look for. Signs or symptoms of Conduct Disorder include:

- Hostility towards people or animals.
- Intimidating harm towards others.
- Frequently starting fights with others.
- Cruelty towards animals.
- Damage of property, such as environment fires.
- Frequently lying.
- Stealing.
- Regular run-ins with regulations.
- Forcing someone into sexual behavior with no person's consent.
- Frequently violating the rights of others.
- Often creating issues by escalating problems.
- Insufficient remorse for bad behavior or hurting

others.
- Difficulty feeling or teaching empathy.
- Breaking into people's homes or cars.
- Conning people.
- Regular attempts to intimidate others.
- Bullying behavior.
- Frequently breaking the rules.
- Getting back in trouble at college frequently.
- Frequently missing school.
- Running abroad.
- Physical fights.
- Viewing others as hostile or aggressive (even though they're not).
- Trouble accurately interpreting public cues.
- Regular injuries from engaging in fights or having accidents.
- Knowing the first steps to take.

In case your observations and instincts cause you to believe your adolescent has Conduct Disorder, the first three steps to consider towards handling the problem are to:

1 - Speak to your teenager: Sit back with your child and communicate your concerns about the troubling behaviors you've observed. You've likely brought these up before, perhaps when you were frustrated or upset. Let your son or daughter know that you would like to assist in any manner you can, which you're willing to pay attention.

Since defiance usually is a significant facet of Conduct Disorder, your child might not be willing to start for you. Don't pressurize, but don't allow yourself to be manipulated either ultimately. You'll need to regularly set firm limitations and anticipations without yelling, lecturing, or engaging in a power struggle.

2 - Setup a scheduled appointment for an assessment: Your child's pediatrician or your loved ones' doctor can be one spot to start. It's essential to keep in mind, however, that he/she isn't a mental doctor with specific training and experience in working with especially challenging disorders like Conduct Disorder. Your physician can execute a physical exam to see whether there's a root medical cause or drug abuse problem that may be leading to or playing a job in your child's behavior.

With Conduct Disorder, it's generally better to have your child evaluated with a psychologist or psychiatrist, ideally a person who specializes in dealing with children and adolescents. Their history and experience allow these professionals to identify and understand the more delicate aspects of Conduct Disorder and the procedure problems associated with it. Ask your loved ones doctor for a recommendation or recommendation.

3 - Get your child into treatment: The 3rd step to consider is to get your child into treatment. The primary form of treatment for Conduct Disorder in teenagers is therapy, although medications enable you to treat co-occurring issues.

Speak Therapy - Three of the very most useful and common types of speak therapy found in the treating

Conduct Disorder include cognitive-behavioural therapy (CBT), multisystemic therapy, behaviour therapy, and family therapy.

Cognitive-behavioural therapy is a kind of talk therapy that targets helping your child identify and change negative thought patterns, self-talk, and beliefs by replacing them with healthy, more positive thoughts, self-talk, and ideas.

- *Multisystemic therapy* can be a rigorous therapy that involves both the family and the city. It can help juvenile offenders by dealing with environmental factors (e.g., home life, educators, friends, community) which may be having an unfortunate effect on your teen.
- *Behaviour therapy* focuses mainly on changing unwanted behaviours using things such as positive reinforcement
- *Family therapy*, particularly *functional family therapy*, targets are identifying and changing harmful family dynamics, which may be adding to or worsening your teen's Conduct Disorder. Useful

family therapy is geared and designed for children who frequently take action out. It targets reducing negativity in the house while increasing support and enhancing communication among families.

Medication - Medication isn't usually used to take care of Conduct Disorder itself. However, it might be recommended to help relieve symptoms of any co-occurring disorders, such as ADHD, stress, or depression. Extreme caution should always be applied as it pertains to medication for children, as their young brains remain developing. However, if your child's symptoms are moderate to severe, the vast benefits usually outweigh the potential risks generally.

Appropriate treatment plans for your son or daughter will be recommended once she or he has been examined.

Assisting and Encouraging Your Child

It could be particularly tricky focusing on how to aid and encourage a teenager with Conduct Disorder, mainly when they're defiant or hostile. Following are some tips:

1. Keep yourself well-informed about Conduct

Disorder so you'll have a much better knowledge of what your child is experiencing and why she or he behaves in specific manners.
2. Speak to your child's therapist or psychiatrist about the easiest way to react to aggressive, destructive, defiant, or cruel behaviors.
3. Set firm boundaries and guidelines in the house, but avoid engaging in power-struggles with your child.
4. Please make yourself available (and prepared) to pay attention and let your child know you're there for her or him.
5. Be reasonable, reasonable, and constant with the guidelines you place and the ways that you enforce them.
6. Communicate guidelines and effects.
7. Be patient, knowing that it will require time for your child to break old patterns of behavior and create a better attitude.
8. Don't take your teen's negative behavior personally.
9. Please encourage your child to use the abilities

they're learning from therapy at home.

10. Understand that Conduct Disorder isn't something your child can merely overcome with sheer willpower; neither is it only a stage of adolescence.

11. Actively take part in your teen's treatment and seek advice from along with his or her treatment provider regarding concerns and questions.

12. Make an effort to create and keep maintaining a low-stress, safe, and structured home environment to help support your teen's treatment and overall emotional health.

13. React to unwanted manners in a company, consistent manner without episode or anger.

14. Strive to keep your cool even if you're frightened or worried.

15. Be genuinely supportive of both your words and actions.

16. Frequently check-in with your son or daughter to observe how they're doing, whether treatment is helping, and also to see when there is whatever you can do this would be helpful.

How to Proceed When Things Escalate

One of the most significant issues of parenting children with Conduct Disorder is that they can be highly impulsive and unpredictable. Because of this, things can quickly escalate and lead to an emergency. If your son or daughter is intimidating to damage or positively harming you or anyone - other families, domestic family pets or other pets, classmates, etc. - then everyone's security is your most significant concern. Turning a blind vision or presuming things will relax independently can result in disastrous outcomes.

If things do escalate, don't delay in reaching out for help. Contact your child's supplier as soon as possible, or, if it's after a few hours;

1. Enlist the assistance of close relatives or friends to work with you.
2. Take your son or daughter to the nearest medical centre (when you can do this safely).

When Individual Therapy isn't enough

Sometimes Individual therapy isn't enough to adequately treat and manage your teen's Conduct Disorder. If your child is:

- Intimidating to, actively likely to, or currently harming another person.
- Threatening or actively planning suicide.
- Making suicide gestures or attempts.
- Struggling to function appropriately at home, school, or other settings.

Then it's time for you to look at a more intensive degree of treatment. This might involve:

Intensive outpatient treatment (IOP) / Psychiatric day treatment

- Residential treatment.
- Dual diagnosis treatment.
- Inpatient psychiatric treatment.
- Rigorous outpatient treatment or psychiatric day treatment may differ in conditions of the quantity of time spent in treatment and exactly how often

(e.g., twice weekly, five days weekly) your son or daughter must go. These programs will be the next thing up from regular outpatient treatment (i.e., one hour of therapy a few times weekly).

- Home treatment involves having your son or daughter stay at a nonhospital treatment facility that specializes in treating adolescents with mental health disorders. Home treatment typically continues between 30 to 180 times, concerning the disease and its severity. If drug abuse is also a problem, choose a home treatment middle that offers dual analysis treatment.

- Dual diagnosis treatment is preferred for adolescents who've both Conduct Disorder and a substance use disorder. This sort of treatment often occurs in a home treatment establishing or within a rigorous outpatient cure.

- Inpatient psychiatric treatment is the best and most rigorous degree of treatment for children who are an imminent danger to themselves or others. It needs admitting your child to a teenager psychiatric hospital device where medical personnel will monitor her or him 24/7. This degree of treatment may last for several days.

Each one of these intensive degrees of treatment typically provides daily therapy in a variety of forms, such as Individual and Group Therapy, and also other types of therapies such as music therapy or artwork therapy. Regular or daily appointments with an employee psychiatrist could also occur, mainly if your child has been treated with medication.

Caring for Yourself

Dealing with a teenager who has Conduct Disorder can elicit a range of negative emotions. These can include emotions of hopelessness, helplessness, anger, disappointment, and despair. You may even struggle with a feeling of failing as a mother or father, blaming yourself for your child's behavior and thinking where you proceeded to go wrong. However, defeating yourself up won't help you, and it really won't benefit your child.

Taking into consideration the emotional toll of Conduct Disorder, you must make a regular, conscientious effort to consider proper care of yourself. Adequate self-care can help prevent those negative feelings from mind-boggling and defeating you and can help bolster your psychological well-being.

Some actions you can take to look after yourself include:

- Encircling yourself with supportive individuals. This might add a therapist, a pastor, or other users of your chapel, local or online organizations, family, and good friends. The more backed up you feel, the simpler it'll be to aid and encourage your child.
- Get plenty of rest and eat a healthy diet plan.
- Make time for yourself.
- Learn healthy ways to control your stress.

Chapter 9

Tantrum

A tantrum is generally a short time of angry outbursts or unreasonable behavior such as crying, screaming, shouting, and throwing items.

What can cause a tantrum?

This is a standard part of growing up. Between your ages of just 1 and four years, most children will have tantrums as children develop, they understand how to become more independent. For instance, they could want to try out, want to dress and give food to themselves or pour their juice. Your son or daughter, therefore, can get very annoyed if they're not able to take action or if they're stopped. A fight between independence and frustration can result in tantrums.

Tantrums can also occur whenever a child is:
- Tired.
- Hungry.

- Feeling ignored.
- Worried or stressed.

A more youthful child may struggle to tell you they are stressed, plus they may cry, become clingy, and also have tantrums.

What may I do when my child is having a Tantrum?

Your son or daughter's screams and yells can be alarming. You might feel upset, discouraged, and hopeless. You will likely be humiliated if a tantrum occurs in a general public place or before other people. It isn't easy being truly a mother or father or carer of the toddler. However, it's essential to set the guidelines, which means that your child discovers to cope with their feelings. Remember, it is common that children will attempt to drive the limits. Below are a few ideas that might do the job as well as your child.

- **Don't panic:**

The crucial thing to do is to remain calm rather than to

get annoyed. Just remind yourself that it is reasonable, a large number of parents do offer with it, be reassured that you'll manage this too.

- **Disregard the tantrum:**

    It would help if you calmly continued with whatever you do - chatting to another person, packaging your shopping, or whatever. Once in a while, check to ensure your son or daughter is safe. Ignoring your son or daughter is very difficult, but if you answer back, or even smack them, you are providing them with interest; they are challenging.

- **Be constant with guidelines:**

    You want to teach your son or daughter that rules are essential and that you'll adhere to them.

- **Focus on any good behavior:**

    Once you see any indicators of calming down - e.g., they stop screaming - compliment them. Change your full attention back again to the kid, speak to them with warmness and admiration. If you incentive the new behavior like this, your son or daughter is much more likely to stay relaxed and keep on being right.

What may I do to avoid temper tantrums?

Planning can help avoid a tantrum if you understand when they will probably happen or notice a design your son or daughter shows before using a tantrum. Below are a few examples:

1. Manage boredom when in a waiting room by firmly taking their favorite books and playthings to the doctor's surgery with you.
2. Keeping their favorite biscuits out of view, rather than where they can easily see them.
3. Manage a tired child, giving them a day nap, rather than staying awake all day long.
4. Manage food cravings by supplying a treat after nursery at 3.30 pm, rather than needing to wait until 5.00 pm for tea.
5. Distraction can help - you might be in a position to avoid a tantrum by diverting your son or daughter's attention.

Where may I get help?

Speaking problems with other parents, family, or friends is often useful. Speak to your child's instructors, as there could be an identical problem at nursery or college.

If this will not help and the tantrums are receiving you down, ask your wellbeing visitor, college, practice nurse, or doctor for advice. Many parents and carers find parenting programs like Triple P or Webster Stratton groupings helpful. Sometimes more expert help from the child and adolescent mental health services (CAMHS) may be needed, mainly when there are other stressing difficulties for the kid, or when tantrums take place too long and frequently, with the kid harming themselves or others.

Chapter 10
Personality Disorders: Helpful Information to the 10 Different Kinds

Individuals who have trouble handling everyday tensions and design of difficulty working with others may have a personality disorder.

Personality disorders are classified by the American Psychiatric Association's Diagnostic and Statistical Manual of Mental Disorders (DSM) as mental ailments and define them. Difficulty dealing with regular stress and trouble developing associations with family, friends, and coworkers may be signs of personality disorder. Those that have a problem with a personality disorder often don't enjoy friendly activities and might not see themselves as adding to their problems. While everyone has its distinctive features, the personality disorders also talk about some typically common characteristics.

"All personality disorders involve a design of behavior that deviates from the expectations of one's culture," says Scott Krakower, DO, associate unit central of psychiatry at Zucker Hillside Medical centre in Glen Oaks, NY. "There could be a distortion in a person's cognition, changes in his effect, or problems getting together with others and perhaps issues with impulse control."

Relating to Mental Health America, personality disorders get into three different categories:

- Cluster A: Odd or eccentric behavior
- Cluster B: Dramatic, emotional or erratic behavior
- Cluster C: Anxious, fearful behavior

While personality disorders may be attentive to treatment, the task is getting the average person with a personality disorder to admit that he has a problem and then consent to treatment. "Many people with personality disorders could reap the benefits of specific therapy," Dr. Krakower says. "However, they may choose never to go for treatment, or they could go only after a considerable worsening of symptoms in an emergency."

People with personality disorders are inclined to comorbid diagnoses like drug abuse disorder, stress, and despair, explains Shawna Newman, MD, a grown-up, child, and adolescent psychiatrist at Lenox Hill Medical center in NEW YORK. "Folks are truly struggling when they have a personality disorder," she says. "Even though their situation can be maintained or managed with treatment, removing a personality disorder can be, at best, very hard and might not be possible." Psychosocial interventions are usually recommended for people that have a personality disorder, but there are no FDA-approved medications to take care of these disorders, Newman clarifies.

When you have an average degree of risk that you'll create a personality disorder if others in your loved ones have one, it's not a given. "Conditions can run in households just like the risk will for diabetes or cardiovascular disease," says John M. Oldham, MD, interim key of personnel at the Menninger Medical centre and Recognized Emeritus Teacher at the Menninger Division of Psychiatry and Behavioral Sciences at the Baylor University of Medication in Texas. "But even though you have risk factors, you might create a personality disorder only when you didn't have balance throughout your early years if there is a disconnection or derailment in the connection process throughout your development."

People that have personality disorders don't own it easy when they remain other folks, Dr. Oldham says. "There's a great deal of stigma, which is true for every mental disorder," he says. "However, we are receiving just a little better about realizing that these are illnesses."
Here, a synopsis of a few of the ten personality disorders outlined in the latest Diagnostic and Statistical Manual of Mental Disorders.

1. ***Borderline Personality Disorder:***
    Is described by the "design of instability in human social relationships, self-image, and impacts, and designated impulsivity," says the DSM. Not merely do they lack a good sense of identification, they have a problem developing and keeping interactions, Dr. Krakower says. However, they could reap the benefits of certain types of therapy such as dialectical behavior therapy (DBT.) DBT

is a cognitive-behavioural treatment that combines person psychotherapy with group skills training classes to help individuals learn new skills and approaches for managing their feelings and reducing the issue in their lives.

Medication can relax the average person, but it's much less useful as psychotherapy, says Dr. Oldham. "If people who have personality disorders find the appropriate therapist, plus they stay with it, there's a good chance they'll progress," he says.

People that have borderline personality disorder are highly concerned that individuals don't like them, Dr. Oldham says. "They could imagine this so vividly that they could start arguing with a person when the individual wasn't even thinking about them," he says. "The person's romantic relationships get rocky because they're so insecure." People with borderline personality disorder tend to be antagonistic and antisocial and could injure themselves by trimming or burning up themselves.

2. Paranoid Personality Disorder:

The average person with this disorder displays distrust toward others that typically starts by early adulthood, Dr. Krakower says. "Furthermore to recurrent suspicions of others, the individual reads concealed meanings into harmless remarks," he points out. "The individual may believe that others are deceiving them." The DSM defines the disorder as "a design of distrust and suspiciousness in a way that other's motives are interpreted as malevolent."

The individual experiencing paranoid personality disorder encounters "suspicion lacking any objective or sufficient basis," says Dr. Newman. "The average person can read negative indicating into very innocent remarks. They perceive a lot of unintentional insults and could be very unforgiving."

3. Schizoid Personality Disorder:

This disorder is "design of detachment from cultural associations and a limited range of psychological appearance," says the DSM. "The individual may become more of the loner and choose solitary activities," Dr. Krakower says. While a person with a schizoid personality disorder can reap the benefits of social skills organizations, unfortunately, they may choose never to look for treatment.

4. *Schizotypal Personality Disorder:*

Is proclaimed by a design of difficulty with human relationships that is followed by cognitive and perceptual distortions and eccentric behaviors, says Dr. Krakower. "The average person may be superstitious and also have magical values or unusual and uncommon ideas," he clarifies. With this disorder, too, as the person could reap the benefits of social skills groupings, they often choose never to look for treatment. People with this disorder are so highly superstitious; these are fundamentally dysfunctional, Dr. Newman says.

"They could have odd values that impact their behavior, such as ideas about clairvoyance or telepathy, and the ones with this personality disorder frequently have very bizarre thoughts," she says. Individuals generally have extreme social panic with everyone except first-degree family members, she says.

5. *Antisocial Personality Disorder:*

This disorder entails the design of behavior that is designated by a disregard for and violation of the privileges of others. They often neglect to conform to public norms, which might lead to repetitive arrests and legal behavior, Dr. Krakower says. "They may end up in prison," he gives. Men with antisocial behavior tend to break regulations, disregard guidelines of conduct, and become manipulative and reckless," says Dr. Oldham. "They show no remorse for the items they do, plus they don't comply with interpersonal norms," he says. "There isn't a good treatment for Antisocial Personality Disorder and you ought to start early in life to attempt to prevent it because once it's there, it's hard to repair."

6. *Histrionic Personality Disorder:*

The individual exhibits a design of attention-seeking behaviors, which might entail an elevated sense of dramatization and improper intimate or provocative practices, Dr. Krakower says. Sometimes, they have Borderline Personality Disorder as well. She could reap the benefits of a kind of therapy known as DBT.

7. *Narcissistic personality disorder:*

This requires a design of grandiose behaviors with an exaggerated sense of personal, Dr. Krakower says. "They are preoccupied with unrealistic images of success and power and could often discover others inferior compared to them," he says.

The person will believe they're special and unique and requires excessive admiration from others, Dr. Oldham says. "They aren't very proficient at having empathy," he says. "Nor are they thinking about trying to comprehend how other folks feel." A person with a narcissistic personality disorder may concurrently have a borderline personality disorder and may benefit from a specific therapy, he says, but regrettably, it's common for the individual to refuse treatment.

8. *An Avoidant Personality Disorder:*
This consists of a design of behavior with heightened sociable inhibition, which is often along with a concern with the rejection of others, Dr. Krakower says. The individual may have emotions of inadequacy and become hypersensitive to negative evaluation, based on the DSM. "With this disorder, generally people might not even recognize that the average person has a personality disorder," says Dr. Oldham. Psychotherapy is the primary treatment, he says.

9. *Reliant Personality Disorder:*
He or she displays a design of behavior proclaimed by extreme neediness or clinginess, followed by

worries of parting, Dr. Krakower says.

10. *Anankastic (Obsessive-Compulsive) Personality Disorder:*

A person with anankastic (obsessive-compulsive) personality disorder shows a design of behavior of extreme orderliness and excellence, Dr. Krakower points out, and he's frequently inflexible and rigid. The average person that has this disorder discovers it difficult to discard items, even if indeed they have little psychological value, he says.

Chapter 11
Avoidant Personality Disorder

A socially uncomfortable person with hypersensitivity to rejection and feelings of inadequacy may have a mental illness known as Avoidant Personality Disorder.

No one likes criticism, rejection, or shame, but sometimes people spend their lifetime staying away from them. A socially challenged person with hypersensitivity to rejection and continuous emotions of inadequacy may have a mental disease known as Avoidant Personality Disorder (AVPD).

People who have Avoidant Personality Disorder experience public awkwardness. They spend lots of time concentrating on their shortcomings and are incredibly hesitant to create interactions where rejection could take place. This often leads to emotions of loneliness and becoming disengaged from romantic relationships at the job and elsewhere. People who have AVPD may also refuse to advertise, make excuses to miss conferences or be too fearful of activating on occasions where they could make friends.

What causes Avoidant Personality Disorder?

Analysts don't wholly know very well what causes avoidance personality disorder; however, they believe that it is a mixture of genetics and environmental factors.

Early childhood encounters may be from the development of AVPD. Research shows that children who see their caregivers as without devotion and encouragement and experience rejection from them may be at increased risk. So can be children who experience mistreatment, neglect, and a standard lower degree of treatment. In response to these encounters, children may avoid socializing with others as a coping strategy.

Researchers think that yet another factor may be experiencing a significant change in appearance thanks to physical disease. Approximately 2.5% of the populace may be eligible for a diagnosis of Avoidant Personality Disorder. It is a chronic disorder that impacts men and women similarly. The disease can form in youth, and symptoms have been recognized in children as young as 24 months old. However, like other personality disorders, Avoidant Personality Disorder usually is only diagnosed in adults.

Avoidant Personality Disorder Symptoms

Avoidant Personality Disorder is seen as comprising of 3 major components:
- Social inhibition.
- Emotions of inadequacy.
- Level of sensitivity to criticism or rejection.

To get an analysis, a person will need to have experienced these components by enough time they reach early adulthood. Besides, they must experience at least four of the following AVPD symptoms:
- Avoidance of activities at the job that involve interpersonal contact thanks to concern with criticism or rejection.
- Unwillingness to connect to others unless sure

they'll get a positive response
- Hesitancy in romantic relationships thanks to concern with shame
- Preoccupation with criticism in sociable situations
- Feeling insufficient and being inhibited in new cultural cases
- Perception of personal as inept, unappealing, and inferior
- Reluctance to take chances or take part in activities that may lead to embarrassment
- A diagnosis will demand a psychological evaluation with a mental doctor. This evaluation will also eliminate other potential diagnoses or determine whether one has several diagnoses.

What is a Cluster C Personality Disorder?

Different personality disorder diagnoses are organized by group, or "cluster." ***Cluster C personality disorders*** are conditions where characteristics involve being especially stressed or fearful. An avoidance personality disorder is a Cluster C personality disorder, as are reliant personality disorder and obsessive-compulsive personality disorder.

Is Avoidant Personality Disorder exactly like Social Anxiety?

Research workers and clinicians used to think that Avoidant Personality Disorder only occurred together with social panic (SAD). However, newer research shows that there surely is a substantial percentage of individuals with AVPD who do not meet up with the criteria for public anxiety disorder.

Sometimes it could be challenging to tell apart whether one has social panic or Avoidant Personality Disorder, or both conditions. Typically, a person with AVPD will experience anxiousness and avoidance in every arena of life, whereas a person with interpersonal anxiety may have worries specific to certain situations, such as presenting and public speaking or performing.

Furthermore, to social panic, individuals with Avoidant Personality Disorder may have co-occurring conditions, including depression, obsessive-compulsive disorder, or other anxiety disorders or personality disorders. People who have AVPD are also at increased threat of drug abuse or suicidal behavior.

Sometimes Avoidant Personality Disorder is also confused with a schizoid personality disorder, as both conditions involve public isolation. However, people with schizoid personality disorder have an over-all disinterest in getting together with others, whereas people who have Avoidant Personality Disorder want associations but have a tendency to avoid them credited to concern with rejection or criticism.

Treatment for Avoidant Personality Disorder

People who have Avoidant Personality Disorder may seek treatment because they would like to build stronger human relationships and decrease the amount of stress they experience at the general public or the job. Dealing with any personality disorder can be difficult, as a person has experienced much of the symptoms for quite some time.

Psychotherapy, or chat therapy, is the first Avoidant Personality Disorder treatment. Psychotherapy can include cognitive-behavioural therapy, which targets reducing negative thought patterns and building sociable skills. Sometimes group therapy can be used to help people who have similar difficulties and produce a safe space to create stable interactions. Family therapy can also show useful so that families understand the problem and can offer a supportive environment that promotes the development and healthy risk-taking.

There is certainly little to no research demonstrating the potency of medication in treating Avoidant Personality Disorder. Sometimes medicines enable you to manage symptoms of Avoidant Personality Disorder or the symptoms of co-occurring disorders. Medications typically include antidepressants (i.e., selective serotonin reuptake inhibitors) and anti-anxiety medications.

Getting Help for Avoidant Personality Disorder

If you have a problem with how never to be socially

awkward and think it's likely you have Avoidant Personality Disorder, it's essential never to be discouraged. Help is available, and the first rung on the ladder is calling your physician or another mental doctor who can conduct an assessment and assess your trouble.

Therapy in a safe and encouraging environment will help you explore the extreme anxiety you have in sociable situations, as well as your concern with rejection or criticism. Collectively, you as well as your therapist can practice challenging negative values and explore the tiny but significant actions you can take to develop solid friendships, become more engaged at the job, and establish romantic relationships with others.

Chapter 12
Antisocial Personality Disorder

Antisocial Personality Disorder describes an ingrained design of behavior where individuals regularly disregard and violate the legal rights of others around them.

The disorder is most beneficially understood within the context of the broader group of personality disorders. A personality disorder can be a long-lasting design of personal experience and behavior that deviates noticeably from the objectives of the individual's culture, is pervasive and inflexible, comes with a starting point in adolescence or early adulthood, is steady as time passes, and leads to personal problems or impairment.

The symptoms of Antisocial Personality Disorder may differ in severity. The greater egregious or dangerous behavior patterns are known as *sociopathic or psychopathic*. There's been much argument regarding the distinction between your two explanations. **Sociopathy** is chiefly characterized as something seriously incorrect with one's conscience; *psychopathy* is portrayed as an entire insufficient conscience regarding others. Some specialists describe people who have this constellation of symptoms as "rock chilly" to the privileges of others — effects of the disorder range from imprisonment, substance abuse, and alcoholism.

People who have this illness may appear charming on the top, but they will tend to be irritable and intense as well as irresponsible. They could have numerous somatic issues as well as perhaps attempt suicide. Because of the manipulative tendencies, it is challenging to inform if they are lying or telling the reality.

The diagnosis of Antisocial Personality Disorder is not directed at individuals under age 18 but is given only when there's a history of some symptoms of Conduct Disorder before age 15. Antisocial Personality Disorder is a lot more prevalent in men than in females. The best prevalence of Antisocial Personality Disorder is available among men who abuse alcoholic beverages or drugs or who are in prisons or other forensic configurations.

Symptoms

Based on the DSM-5, top features of Antisocial Personality Disorder include:
- Violation of the physical or emotional privileges of others.
- Lack of balance in the job and home life.
- Irritability and aggression.
- Insufficient remorse.
- Consistent irresponsibility.
- Recklessness, impulsivity.
- Deceitfulness.

A year as a child diagnosis (or symptoms constant with) Conduct Disorder

A mental evaluation verifies an antisocial personality. Other disorders should be eliminated first, as this is a significant diagnosis.

The alcohol and substance abuse common among people who have Antisocial Personality Disorder can exacerbate symptoms of the disorder. When drug abuse and

Antisocial Personality Disorder coexist, treatment is more difficult for both.

Causes

As the specific factors behind the disorder are unknown, both environmental and genetic factors have been implicated. Hereditary factors are suspected because the occurrence of antisocial behavior is higher in people who have a biological mother or father who shows antisocial characteristics. Environmental factors could also are likely involved; however, as a person whose role model experienced antisocial tendencies is much more likely to build up to them.
About 3% of men and about 1% of women have Antisocial Personality Disorder.

Treatment

Treatment for Antisocial Personality Disorder may prove challenging. As the symptoms of the disorder tend to maximize in a person's early 20s, people could find that symptoms improve independently as a person gets to their 40s and beyond.

Psychotherapy, or chat therapy, is usually the procedure recommended for Antisocial Personality Disorder. A therapist can help a person manage negative behaviors and build social skills they could lack. Often the first goal is merely to lessen impulsive habits that can result in arrest or physical damage. Family therapy might be considered a useful option to teach family and improve communication, and group therapy also may help when limited by people who have the disorder.

No medications have been approved by the U.S. Food and Medication Administration to take care of Antisocial Personality Disorder. Vaccination may sometimes be recommended in reducing intense or impulsive behaviors. Medications might include disposition stabilizers or antidepressants.

Treatment also needs to address any co-occurring disorders, which frequently include attention-deficit/hyperactivity disorder, borderline personality disorder, and impulse control disorders such as gaming disorder or sexual disorders. Just because a majority of individuals with Antisocial Personality Disorder will likewise have a drug abuse disorder, a person might need to complete cleansing as the first rung on the ladder of treatment, with the drug abuse and personality disorder then treated concurrently.

Antisocial Personality Disorder is one of the very most difficult personality disorders to take care of. Individuals hardly ever seek treatment independently and may start therapy only once mandated to take action by a courtroom. There is no indicated treatment for Antisocial Personality Disorder. Lately, the antipsychotic medication clozapine shows promising leads to enhancing symptoms among men with Antisocial Personality Disorder.

At what Age can Antisocial Personality Disorder be Diagnosed?

A person must be at least 18 years of age to get an analysis of Antisocial Personality Disorder. There must be proof that they certified for a medical diagnosis of Conduct Disorder before the age group of 15, as much of the symptoms of both disorders are similar. An analysis of Antisocial Personality Disorder will also not get if the behaviors happen because of the symptoms of schizophrenia or bipolar disorder.

How to Cope whenever a Cherished One has Antisocial Personality Disorder

When you have someone you care about with antisocial personality, it's common to feel discouraged. Keeping in mind that insufficient remorse or empathy is an indicator of the problem will help you arranged realistic targets for how your beloved can improve. With treatment, many people with Antisocial Personality Disorder do figure out how to form positive romantic relationships, be more accountable, and respect the limitations of others. Others won't, and family must consider how they would like to react to this problem. One interesting simple truth is that individuals with Antisocial Personality Disorder who are wedded tend to improve as time passes compared to one people.

When you have someone you care about with Antisocial Personality Disorder, ensure that additionally, you prioritize your health insurance and safety-family people often think it is useful to take part individual guidance themselves to help manage feelings and figure out how to collection appropriate limitations with the relative.

If you believe it's likely you have Antisocial Personality Disorder or have someone you care about would you, don't hesitate to attain out to your physician or a mental doctor. They can offer information and connect you with the right resources to help you deal with this problem.

Chapter 13
Oppositional Defiant Disorder

What's Oppositional Defiant Disorder (ODD)?

ODD is a behavior disorder, usually diagnosed in child years, that is seen as uncooperative, defiant, negativistic, irritable, and annoying actions toward parents, peers, educators, and other specialist statistics. Children with ODD are more distressing or troubling to others than these are distressed or stressed themselves.

What can cause Oppositional Defiant Disorder?

While the reason behind ODD is as yet not known, there are two primary theories needed to explain the introduction of ODD. A developmental approach shows that problems start when children are small children. Children who develop ODD may experience a hard time understanding how to separate and be autonomous from the principal person to whom these were psychologically attached. The "bad behavior" characteristics of ODD are seen as a continuation of the standard developmental conditions that were not adequately resolved through the toddler years. Learning theory suggests, however, that the negativistic characteristics of ODD are discovered attitudes, reflecting the consequences of negative encouragement techniques utilized by parents and power figures. The usage of negative support by parents can be regarded as increasing the pace and strength of oppositional behaviors in the kid as it achieves the required attention, time, concern, and conversation with parents or expert figures.

Who is suffering from Oppositional Defiant Disorder?
Behavior disorders are, undoubtedly, the most typical reason for recommendations to mental health services for children. Oppositional Defiant Disorder is reported to impact 1% to 16% of the school-age populace. ODD is more prevalent in young boys than in young ladies.

What are the symptoms of Oppositional Defiant Disorder?

Most symptoms observed in children with Oppositional Defiant Disorder also occur sometimes in children without this disorder, especially around the age range or two or three 3, or through the teenage years. Many children, especially when they are exhausted, hungry, or annoyed, tend to disobey, argue with parents, or defy specialists. However, in children with Oppositional Defiant Disorder, these symptoms take place more often and hinder learning, school modification, and, sometimes, with the child's romantic relationships with others.

Symptoms of Oppositional Defiant Disorder can include:
- Regular temper tantrums.
- Extreme arguments with adults.
- Refusal to adhere to adult requests.
- Always questioning guidelines; refusal to check out rules.

- Behavior designed to annoy or annoying others, including adults.
- Blaming others for your misbehaviors or mistakes.
- Easily frustrated by others.
- Frequently having an angry attitude.
- Speaking harshly or unkindly.
- Seeking revenge

The symptoms of ODD look like other medical ailments or behavior problems. Always seek advice from your child's doctor for an analysis.

How is Oppositional Defiant Disorder Diagnosed?

Parents, instructors, and other power numbers in child and adolescent configurations often identify the kid or adolescent with ODD. However, a kid psychiatrist or a professional mental doctor usually diagnoses ODD in children. A detailed background of the child's behavior from parents and educators, medical observations of the child's behavior, and, sometimes, mental testing donate to the medical diagnosis. Parents who take note of symptoms of ODD in the youngster or teenager can help by seeking an assessment and treatment early. Early treatment could prevent future problems.

Further, Oppositional Defiant Disorder often coexists with other mental health disorders, including feeling disorders, anxiety disorders, Conduct Disorder, and attention-deficit/hyperactivity disorder, increasing the necessity for early analysis and treatment. Check with your child's doctor to find out more.

Treatment for Oppositional Defiant Disorder

Specific treatment for children with Oppositional Defiant Disorder will be dependent on your child's doctor predicated on:

- Your son or daughter's age, general health, and health background.
- The extent of your son or daughter's symptoms.
- Your son or daughter's tolerance for specific

medications or therapies.
- Objectives for the span of the condition.
- Your opinion or preference.

Treatment can include:
- **Individual psychotherapy:** Person psychotherapy for ODD often uses cognitive-behavioural methods to improve problem resolving skills, communication skills, impulse control, and anger management skills.
- **Family therapy:** Family therapy is often centred on making changes within the family system, such as enhancing communication skills and family relationships. Parenting children with ODD can be quite tricky and attempting for parents. Parents need support and understanding as well as assist in developing far better parenting approaches.
- **Peer group therapy:** Peer group therapy is often centred on developing sociable skills and social skills.
- **Medication:** Without considered effective in dealing with ODD, medication can be utilized if

other symptoms or disorders can be found and attentive to medication.

Avoidance of Oppositional Defiant Disorder in Children

Some experts think that a developmental series of encounters occur in the introduction of Oppositional Defiant Disorder. This series may begin with inadequate parenting practices, accompanied by difficulty with other expert statistics and poor peer connections. As these encounter substance and continue, oppositional and defiant behaviors turn into a design of action.

Early recognition and involvement in negative family and cultural encounters may help disrupt the series of experiences resulting in more oppositional and defiant behaviors. Early identification and treatment with an increase of practical communication skills, parenting skills, discord quality skills, and anger management skills can disrupt the design of negative behaviors and reduce the disturbance of oppositional and defiant behaviors in social associations with adults and peers, and college and social modification.

The purpose of early treatment is to improve the child's healthy development and development and enhance the standard of living experienced by children with Oppositional Defiant Disorder.

Chapter 14
Disruptive Behaviour Disorders

Disruptive Behavior Disorders are among easy and straightforward to identify of most coexisting conditions because they involve behaviors that are readily seen, such as temper tantrums, physical aggression such as attacking other children, extreme argumentativeness, stealing, and different kinds of defiance or resistance to authority. These disorders, such as ODD and Conduct Disorder, often first appeal to notice when they hinder college performance or family and peer human relationships, and sometimes intensify as time passes.

Behaviors typical of Disruptive Behavior Disorders can closely resemble ADHD-particularly where impulsivity and hyperactivity are involved-but ADHD, ODD, and Conduct Disorder is considered specific conditions that may appear independently. About 1/3 of most children with ADHD have coexisting ODD, or more to one fourth have coexisting Conduct Disorder. Children with both conditions generally have more challenging lives than people that have ADHD only because their defiant behavior leads to so many issues with adults as well as others with whom they interact. Early recognition and treatment may, however, boost the chances that your son or daughter can figure out how to control these manners.

Oppositional Defiant Disorder

Many children with ADHD display oppositional behaviors sometimes. Oppositional Defiant Disorder is described in the American Psychiatric Association's Diagnostic and Statistical Manual of Mental Disorders, 4th Release (DSM-IV) as including prolonged symptoms of "negativistic, defiant, disobedient, and hostile behaviors toward specialist figures." A kid with ODD may frequently claim with adults, lose his temper quickly; won't follow guidelines; blame others for his errors, intentionally annoy others, and normally behave in furious, resentful, and cruel ways. He's more likely to encounter regular social issues and disciplinary situations at college. Frequently, especially without early medical diagnosis and treatment, these symptoms get worse over time-sometimes becoming severe enough to lead to a medical diagnosis of Conduct Disorder eventually.

Conduct Disorder is a far more extreme condition than ODD. Described in the DSM-IV as "a repeated and persistent design of behavior where the basic privileges of others or major age group appropriate social guidelines are violated," Conduct Disorder may involve serious hostility toward people or the harming of pets, deliberate devastation of property (vandalism), stealing, operating abroad, skipping college, or otherwise wanting to break a few of the significant guidelines of culture without getting captured. Many children with Conduct Disorder were or might have been identified as having ODD at a youthful age-particularly those who have been physically intense when these were more youthful. As the Conduct Disorder symptoms become apparent, these children usually maintain their ODD symptoms (argumentativeness, level of resistance, etc.) as well. This cluster of behaviors, combined with impulsiveness and hyperactivity of ADHD, sometimes causes these children to be looked at as delinquents, and they're apt to be suspended from college and also have more law enforcement contact than children with ADHD by itself or ADHD with ODD.

Children with ADHD whose Conduct Disorder symptoms started young also tend to fare more poorly in adulthood than people that have ADHD only or ADHD with ODD-particularly in the regions of delinquency, unlawful behavior, and drug abuse.

ODD and Conduct Disorder: What things to look for

A kid with ADHD and a coexisting disruptive behavior disorder may very well be much like children with ADHD by itself in conditions of intelligence, health background, and neurological development. He's probably kind of impulsive than children with ADHD only, although if he has Conduct Disorder, his educators or other adults may misinterpret his intense behavior as ADHD-type impulsiveness.
(Attention-deficit/hyperactivity disorder behavior without Conduct Disorder, however, will not typically involve

this degree of hostility.) A kid with ADHD and Conduct Disorder does have a more significant potential for experiencing learning disabilities such as reading disorders and verbal impairment. However, what distinguishes children with ODD and Conduct Disorder most from children with ADHD only is their defiant, resistant, even (regarding CD) intense, cruel, or delinquent behavior.

Other signals to consider include:

- **Family members with ADHD/ODD, ADHD/Conduct Disorder, and Depressive Disorder panic:**

    A kid with a family with ADHD/ODD or ADHD/Conduct Disorder should be viewed for ADHD/Conduct Disorder as well. The likelihood of developing Conduct Disorder is also higher if the family has observed depressive, nervousness, or learning disorders.

- **Stress or turmoil in the family**:

Divorce, parting, drug abuse, parental legal activity, or severe issues within the family are prevalent amongst children with ADHD and coexisting ODD or Conduct

Disorder.

- **Poor or no positive response to the behaviour therapy techniques at home with school:**
  If your son or daughter defies your instructions, violates time-out methods, and otherwise won't cooperate with your use of appropriate behavior therapy techniques, and his intense behavior proceeds unabated, he should be examined for coexisting ODD or Conduct Disorder.

Treatment

Children with ADHD and Disruptive Behavior Disorders often reap the benefits of special behavioral techniques that may be implemented at home with college. These methods typically include options for training your son or daughter to be more alert to his anger cues, use these cues as indicators to start various coping strategies ("Take five deep breaths and take into account the three best options for how to react before lashing out at an instructor."), and offer himself with positive encouragement (informing himself, "Good job, you caught the transmission and used your strategies!") for successful self-control. You as well as your child's instructors, meanwhile, can figure out how to better manage ODD or CD-type behavior through negotiating, diminishing, problem-solving with your son or daughter, anticipating and staying away from possibly explosive situations, and prioritizing goals so that less critical problems are disregarded until more pressing issues have been adequately resolved. Professional behavior therapists can train these highly specific techniques, or other mental medical researchers recommended by your child's pediatrician or college psychologist or other experts associated with your family.

If your son or daughter has a diagnosis of coexisting ODD or CD, and well-planned classroom behavioral techniques in his mainstream classroom have been ineffective, this might lead to a choice to put him in a particular class at school that is established to get more intensive behavior management. However, colleges are mandated to teach your son or daughter in a mainstream classroom if possible, and also to regularly review your child's education plan and reassess the appropriateness of his positioning.

There is recurring evidence that the same stimulant medications that enhance the primary ADHD symptoms also may help to coexist ODD and CD. Stimulants have been proven to help lower verbal and physical hostility, negative peer relationships, stealing, and vandalism. Although stimulant medications do not train children new skills, such as assisting them in identifying and reacting appropriately to others' interpersonal signals, they could decrease the hostility that stands in the form of forming interactions with others how old they are. Because of this, stimulants are usually the first choice in a medication remedy approach for children with ADHD and a coexisting disruptive behavior disorder.

The sooner stimulants are introduced to take care of coexisting ODD or CD, the better. A kid with a disruptive behavior disorder whose intense behavior proceeds untreated may begin to identify with other people who experience self-discipline problems. By adolescence, he might withstand treatment that may help him change his behavior and make him less well-liked by these friends. He'll have grown familiar with his defiant "self" and feel unpleasant and "unreal" when stimulants help check his reckless, authority-flaunting style. By dealing with these behaviors in the first college or even previously, you might have a better potential for preventing your son or daughter from creating a poor self-identity.

If your son or daughter has been treated with two or even more types of stimulants and his aggressive symptoms will be the same or worse, his paediatrician might want to reevaluate the problem and replace the tonic with other medications. If stimulant vaccination by itself resulted in some, however, not enough improvement, his paediatrician may continue steadily to prescribe stimulants in the mixture, essential other agents.

www.ingramcontent.com/pod-product-compliance
Lightning Source LLC
Chambersburg PA
CBHW071109030426
42336CB00013BA/2013